KETO SLOW C

RECIPES

50+ HEALTHY AND EASY LOW-CARB
KETOGENIC RECIPES THAT COOK
BY THEMSELVES IN YOUR CROCKPOT.
LOSE WEIGHT WITH TASTE.

Mary Food

TABLE OF CONTENT

Introduction

The ketogenic diet is a meal plan that will help you to lose weight quickly and without too much effort. It also has the advantage of preventing allergic reactions, mood swings, irritability, fatigue, fat around the waist, heart attacks, decreases the level of bad cholesterol and also it helps to improve your mental capacity.

The ketogenic diet may be helpful for people with metabolic syndrome; it may help with weight loss and lower cholesterol levels. The principle of this diet is to induce a state of ketosis. This entails that you should have an elevated level of ketones in your bloodstream. These ketones your body produces are responsible for turning your body into fat burning mode. Similar to when you are fasting, your body turns fat into ketones. When you are on the ketogenic diet, you will therefore force your body to burn fat. You are basically tricking your system into thinking you are fasting.

One of the reasons why many people are overweight is because they eat too many carbohydrates. Carbohydrates have a strong effect on insulin release. That is why too many of them will cause an increase in body fat levels. Consuming carbohydrates also causes a release of insulin, which in turn will cause the blood sugar levels to dip. When they dip, brain sends out signals that will cause your sugar levels to return to normal. That is how carbohydrates are able to cause weight gain as your body will store the extra sugar as fat.

This is the reason why it is very important for you to avoid them. When you go through intermittent periods of fasting (as in the Atkins diet), you will also be able to kick start your weight loss. When your body starts to get used to not having all those carbohydrates in your bloodstream, it will begin to burn fat for energy. This will help to reduce the fat in your body and your risk of many serious diseases.

If you want to lose weight and improve your health, the first thing you should do is to try out this diet and stick to it. You will be able to lose weight quickly and also help to avoid many chronic diseases. You will also notice that your mood will improve along with your libido. Over time you should see a reduction of fat around your waist and you will also see a big improvement in your mental capacity. If you are interested in losing weight and improving your health, you should begin the ketogenic diet.

What is slow cooking?

Slow cooking is defined as a method in which several ingredients are cooked together at low temperatures for a long time. Slow cooking can also help retain texture, together with moisture and taste. Slow cooking is commonly used in huge cuts like pork shoulder or pork leg. Pork shoulder normally takes 16 hours to cook before it will be ready. However, with a slow cooker, you are able to cook it in 10 hours or less. Using a slow cooker to cook meat gives meat a very rich flavor and tenderness. In slow cooking, meat cooks slowly and the pieces are also cut a bit thicker. The pieces are seared slightly and tenderize in their juices. They are then submerged in the juices at the bottom of the slow cooker. Another interesting tidbit about slow cooking is that some ingredients can leave meat during the process of slow cooking, like carrots, onion, celery, and tarragon, as well as garlic. These then flavor the final preparation.

Slow cooking can be used to make dishes like soups, stews, roasts, and steaks. These dishes will be very tender and tasty when finished. To sum up, slow cooking is the process of preparing dishes in a long, covered cooking pot, usually maintaining low temperatures. It is an excellent way to cook meat until it is extremely delicious and tender.

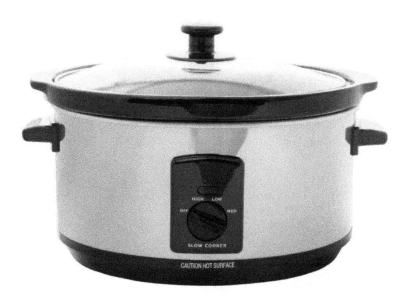

Breakfast

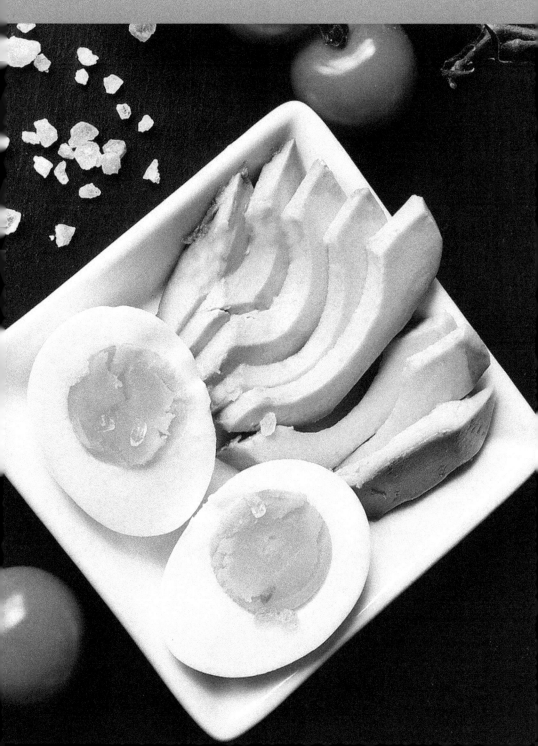

Egg Sausage Breakfast Casserole

Preparation Time: 10 minutes

Cooking Time: 4 hours

Servings: 6

Ingredients:

- 4 cups broccoli, chopped
- 10 eggs
- 1 cup cheddar cheese, shredded
- 12 oz. sausage, cooked and sliced
- ¾ cup whipping cream
- Pepper and salt

Directions:

1. Spray slow cooker from inside with cooking spray.
2. Add half broccoli florets to the slow cooker and spread well.
3. Add ½ sausages and ½ cheeses into the slow cooker.
4. Repeat same with remaining broccoli florets, sausage, and cheese.
5. In a bowl, whisk together eggs, pepper, whipping cream, and salt. Pour into the slow cooker.
6. Cover slow cooker with lid and cook on low for 4 hours.
7. Serve warm and enjoy.

Nutrition:

- Calories 437 Fat 34.5 g Carbs 5.3 g Sugar 1.7 g Protein 27 g Cholesterol 357 mg

Vegetable Omelet

Preparation Time: 10 minutes

Cooking Time: 1 hour 30 minutes

Servings: 4

Ingredients:

- 6 eggs
- 1 bell pepper, diced
- 1 cup spinach
- ½ cup unsweetened almond milk
- 4 egg whites
- Pepper and salt

Directions:

1. Spray slow cooker from inside with cooking spray.
2. In a large bowl, whisk together egg whites, eggs, almond milk, pepper, and salt. Stir in bell pepper and spinach.

3. Transfer egg mixture to the slow cooker.

4. Cover slow cooker with lid and cook on high for 1 hour 30 minutes.

5. Slice and serve.

Nutrition:

- Calories 128 Fat 7.2 g Carbs 3.5 g Sugar 2.3 g Protein 12.5 g Cholesterol 246 mg

Cheese Bacon Quiche

Preparation Time: 10 minutes

Cooking Time: 4 hours

Servings: 8

Ingredients:

- 10 eggs, beaten
- 10 bacon pieces, cooked and chopped
- 8 oz. cheddar cheese, shredded
- 1 cup half and half
- ½ cup spinach, chopped
- Pepper and salt

Directions:

1. Spray slow cooker from inside with cooking spray.
2. In a bowl, whisk together eggs, spinach, cheese, half and half, pepper, and salt.
3. Pour egg mixture into the slow cooker. Sprinkle bacon on top.
4. Cover slow cooker with lid and cook on low for 4 hours.
5. Slice and serve.

Nutrition:

- Calories 252 Fat 20.2 g Carbs 2.6 g Sugar 0.6 g Protein 15.6 g Cholesterol 246 mg

Egg Breakfast Casserole

Preparation Time: 10 minutes

Cooking Time: 1 hour 30 minutes

Servings: 4

Ingredients:

- 6 eggs
- 1 cup cheese, shredded
- 1 lb. ham, chopped into cubes
- 2 green onions, chopped

- ½ cup heavy cream
- Pepper and salt

Directions:

1. Spray slow cooker from inside with cooking spray.
2. In a bowl, whisk together eggs and heavy cream. Add green onions and ham to the bowl and stir well.
3. Pour egg mixture into the slow cooker. Add cheese and black pepper. Stir to mix.
4. Cover slow cooker with lid and cook on high for 1 hour.
5. Stir well and cook for 30 minutes more.
6. Serve warm and enjoy.

Nutrition:

- Calories 447 Fat 31.2 g Carbs 6.2 g Sugar 0.9 g Protein 34.6 g Cholesterol 360 mg

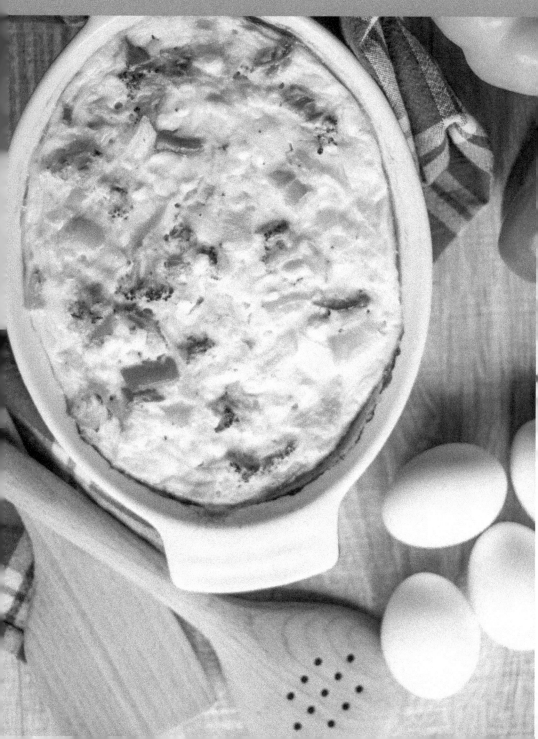

Cauliflower Mashed

Preparation Time: 10 minutes

Cooking Time: 6 hours

Servings: 4

Ingredients:

- 1 medium cauliflower head, cut into florets
- 2 garlic cloves, minced
- 1 ½ cups water
- Pepper and salt

Directions:

1. Add cauliflower florets, garlic, and water into the slow cooker.
2. Cover slow cooker with lid and cook on low for 6 hours.
3. Drain cauliflower well and transfer into the large bowl.
4. Mash cauliflower using the potato masher until smooth and creamy.
5. Season with pepper and salt.
6. Stir well and serve warm.

Nutrition:

- Calories 38 Fat 0.2 g Carbs 8.1 g Sugar 3.5 g Protein 3 g Cholesterol 0 mg

Pork Tenderloin

Preparation Time: 10 minutes

Cooking Time: 4 hours

Servings: 6

Ingredients:

- 1 ½ lbs. pork tenderloin, trimmed and cut in half lengthwise
- 6 garlic cloves, chopped
- 1 oz. envelope dry onion soup mix
- ¾ cup red wine
- 1 cup water
- Pepper and salt

Directions:

1. Place pork tenderloin into the slow cooker.
2. Pour red wine and water over pork.
3. Sprinkle dry onion soup mix on top of pork tenderloin.
4. Top with chopped garlic and season with pepper and salt.
5. Cover slow cooker with lid and cook on low for 4 hours.
6. Stir well and serve.

Nutrition:

- Calories 196 Fat 4 g Carbs 3.1 g Sugar 0.9 g Protein 29.9 g Cholesterol 83 mg

Italian Frittata

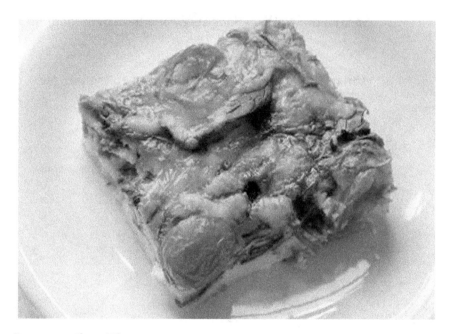

Preparation Time: 10 minutes

Cooking Time: 4 hours

Servings: 4

Ingredients:

- 6 eggs
- 1/4 cup cherry tomatoes, sliced

- 4 oz. mushrooms, sliced
- 2 tsp. Italian seasoning
- 1/2 cup cheddar cheese, shredded
- Pepper
- Salt

Directions:

1. Spray a crock pot inside with cooking spray.
2. Spray a pan with cooking spray and heat over medium heat.
3. Add mushrooms and cherry tomatoes to the pan and cook until softened.
4. Transfer vegetables to the crock pot.
5. In a bowl, whisk together eggs, cheese, pepper, and salt.
6. Pour egg mixture in the crock pot.
7. Cover and cook on low for 4 hours.
8. Slice and serve.

Nutrition:

- Calories 167 Fat 12 g Carbs 2.3 g Sugar 1.6 g Protein 12.8 g Cholesterol 262 mg

Cauliflower Casserole

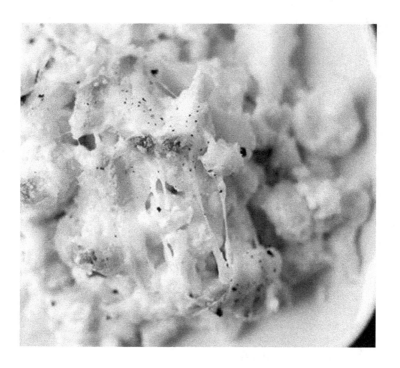

Preparation Time: 10 minutes

Cooking Time: 6 hours

Servings: 8

Ingredients:

- 12 eggs
- 1/2 cup unsweetened almond milk
- 1 lb. sausage, cooked and crumbled
- 1 cauliflower head, shredded
- 2 cups cheddar cheese, shredded

- Pepper
- Salt

Directions:

1. Spray a crock pot inside with cooking spray.
2. In a bowl, whisk together eggs, almond milk, pepper, and salt.
3. Add about a third of the shredded cauliflower into the bottom of the crock pot. Season with pepper and salt.
4. Top with about a third of the sausage and a third of the cheese.
5. Repeat the same layers 2 more times.
6. Pour egg mixture into the crock pot.
7. Cover and cook on low for 6 hours.
8. Serve and enjoy.

Nutrition:

- Calories 443 Fat 35.6 g Carbs 3.5 g Sugar 2 g Protein 27.4 g Cholesterol 323 mg

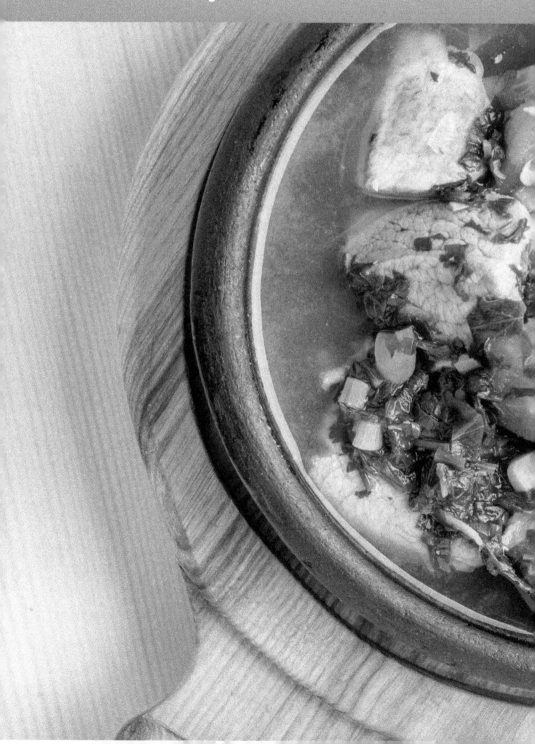

Soups & Stews

Herbed Chicken & Green Chiles Soup

Preparation Time: 15 minutes

Cooking Time: 6 Hours

Servings: 8 (13.1 Ounces per Serving)

Ingredients:

- 2 chicken breasts, boneless, skinless

- ½ teaspoon cumin, ground

- 1 teaspoon onion powder

- 1 teaspoon chili powder

- 1 teaspoon garlic powder

- ½ teaspoon white pepper, ground

- ¼ teaspoon cayenne pepper

- 4 ounces green chilies

- 3 cups water

- ½ avocado, cubed

- 2 tablespoons extra virgin olive oil

Directions:

1. Grease the bottom of Crock-Pot with olive oil and place chicken inside pot.

2. Mix white pepper, cumin, garlic, onion, and chili powder.

3. Sprinkle evenly over the chicken. Place the chilies on top of chicken.

4. Pour in water and stir. Close the lid and cook on HIGH for an hour.

5. Open the lid and give a good stir. Close the lid and continue to cook on HIGH for 5 hours.

6. Serve hot with avocado.

Nutrition:

- Calories 180.02 Total Fat 7.04 g Saturated Fat 1.19 g Cholesterol 18.28 mg

  Sodium 831.99 mg Potassium 599.6 mg Total Carbs 9.82 g Fiber 3.93 g Sugar 1.6 g Protein 13.02 g

Butternut Squash Soup

Preparation Time: 15 minutes

Cooking Time: 7 Hours

Servings: 5

Ingredients:

- 2 cups butternut squash, chopped
- 3 cups chicken stock
- 1 cup heavy cream
- 1 teaspoon ground cardamom
- 1 teaspoon ground cinnamon

Directions:

1. Put the butternut squash in the Slow Cooker.
2. Sprinkle it with ground cardamom and ground cinnamon.
3. Then add chicken stock.
4. Close the lid and cook the soup on High for 5 hours.
5. Then blend the soup until smooth with the help of the immersion blender and add heavy cream.
6. Cook the soup on high for 2 hours more.

Nutrition:

- Calories 125 Protein 1.7g Carbs 7.5g Fat 9.3g Fiber 2g
  Cholesterol 33mg

  Sodium 485mg Potassium 301mg

Turmeric Squash Soup

Preparation Time: 15 minutes

Cooking Time: 9 Hours

Servings: 6

Ingredients:

- 3 chicken thighs, skinless, boneless, chopped

- 3 cups butternut squash, chopped

- 1 teaspoon ground turmeric

- 1 onion, sliced

- 1 oz. green chilies, chopped, canned

- 6 cups of water

Directions:

1. Put chicken thighs in the bottom of the Slow Cooker and
   top them with green chilies.

2.   Then add the ground turmeric, butternut squash, and water.   Add sliced onion and close the lid.

3.   Cook the soup on low for 9 Hours.

Nutrition:

- Calories 194 Protein 22.6g Carbs 8.4g Fat 5.8g Fiber 3.2g Cholesterol 65mg

  Sodium 78mg Potassium 551mg

Sides

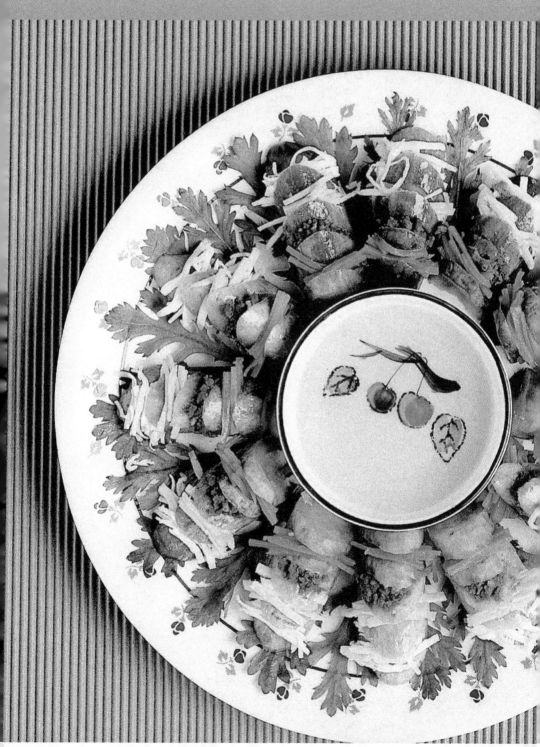

Marjoram Rice Mix

Preparation Time: 15 minutes

Cooking Time: 6 Hours

Servings: 2

Ingredients:

- 1 cup cauliflower rice
- 2 cups chicken stock
- 2 tablespoons marjoram, chopped
- 1 tablespoon olive oil
- A pinch of salt and black pepper
- 1 tablespoon green onions, chopped

Directions:

1. In your Crock Pot, mix the rice with the stock and after that add the other ingredients, toss, put the lid on and cook on Low for 6 hours.
2. Divide between plates and serve.

Nutrition:

- Calories 200 Fat 2 g Fiber 3 g Carbs 7 g Protein 5 g

Cabbage and Onion Mix

Preparation Time: 15 minutes

Cooking Time: 2 Hours

Servings: 2

Ingredients:

- 1 and ½ cups green cabbage, shredded
- 1 cup red cabbage, shredded
- 1 tablespoon olive oil
- 1 red onion, sliced
- 2 spring onions, chopped
- ½ cup tomato paste
- ¼ cup veggie stock
- 2 tomatoes, chopped
- 2 jalapenos, chopped
- 1 tablespoon chili powder
- 1 tablespoon chives, chopped
- A pinch of salt and black pepper

Directions:

1. Grease your Crock Pot with the oil and mix the cabbage with the onion, spring onions and the other ingredients inside.
2. Toss, put the lid on and cook on High for hours.
3. Divide between plates and serve as a side dish.

Cauliflower Mix

Preparation Time: 15 minutes

Cooking Time: 4 Hours

Servings: 2

Ingredients:

- 1 cup cauliflower florets
- 1 cup veggie stock
- ½ cup tomato sauce
- 1 tablespoon chives, chopped
- Salt and black pepper to the taste
- 1 teaspoon sweet paprika

Directions:

1. In your Crock Pot, mix the cauliflower, stock and the other ingredients, toss, put the lid on and cook on High for 4 hours.
2. Divide between plates and serve as a side dish.

Nutrition:

- Calories 135 Fat 5 g Fiber 1 g Carbs 7 g Protein 3 g

Broccoli Mix

Preparation Time: 15 minutes

Cooking Time: 2 Hours

Servings: 10

Ingredients:

- 6 cups broccoli florets
- 1 and ½ cups cheddar cheese, shredded
- 10 ounces canned cream of celery soup
- ½ teaspoon Worcestershire sauce
- ¼ cup yellow onion, chopped
- Salt and black pepper to the taste
- 1 cup crackers, crushed
- 2 tablespoons soft butter

Directions:

1. In a bowl, mix broccoli with cream of celery soup, cheese, salt, pepper, onion and Worcestershire sauce, toss and transfer to your Crock Pot.
2. Add butter, toss again, sprinkle crackers, cover and cook on High for hours.
3. Serve as a side dish.

Nutrition:

- Calories 159 Fat 11 g Fiber 1 g Carbs 11 g Protein 6 g

Roasted Beets

Preparation Time: 15 minutes

Cooking Time: 4 Hours

Servings: 5

Ingredients:

- 10 small beets
- 5 teaspoons olive oil
- A pinch of salt and black pepper

Directions:

1. Divide each beet on a tin foil piece, drizzle oil, season them with salt and pepper, rub well, wrap beets, place them in your Crock Pot, cover and cook on High for 4 hours.
2. Unwrap beets, cool them down a bit, peel, and slice and serve them as a side dish.

Nutrition:

- Calories 100 Fat 2 g Fiber 2 g Carbs 4 g Protein 5 g

Snacks & Appetizers

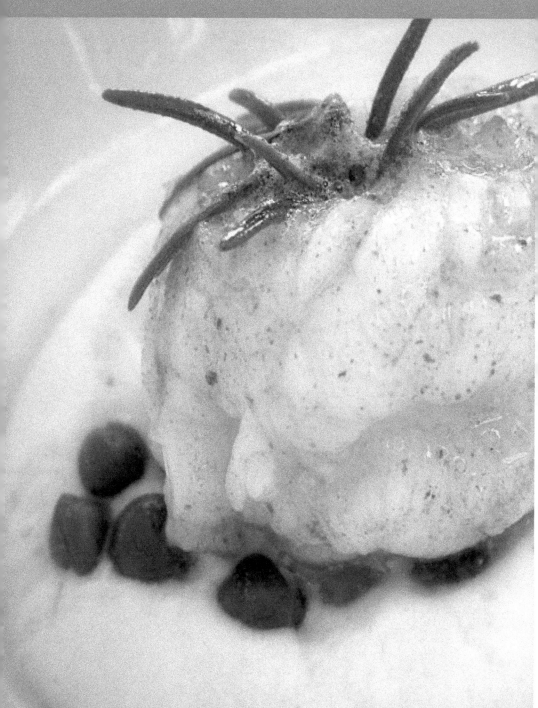

Spicy Pecans

Preparation Time: 10 minutes

Cooking Time: 3 hours

Servings: 16

Ingredients:

- 3 lbs. pecan halves

- 2 tbsp. Cajun seasoning blend

- 2 tbsp. olive oil

Directions:

1. Add all ingredients to the slow cooker and stir well to combine.

2. Cover slow cooker with lid and cook on low for 1 hour.

3. Stir well. Cover again and cook for 2 hours more.

4. Serve and enjoy.

Nutrition:

- Calories 607 Fat 62.5 g Carbs 12.2 g Sugar 3 g Protein 9.1 g Cholesterol 0 mg

Tasty Seasoned Mixed Nuts

Preparation Time: 10 minutes

Cooking Time: 2 hours

Servings: 20

Ingredients:

- 8 cups mixed nuts
- 3 tbsp. curry powder
- 4 tbsp. butter, melted
- Salt

Directions:

1. Add all ingredients into the slow cooker and stir well to combine.
2. Cover slow cooker with lid and cook on high for a ½ hour. Stir again and cook for 30 minutes more.
3. Cover again and cook on low for 1 hour more.
4. Stir well and serve.

Nutrition:

- Calories 375 Fat 34.7 g Carbs 12.8 g Sugar 2.5 g Protein 9 g Cholesterol 6 mg

Nacho Cheese Dip

Preparation Time: 10 minutes

Cooking Time: 2 hours

Servings: 8

Ingredients:

- 8 oz. cream cheese, cut into chunks

- ¼ cup almond milk

- ½ cup chunky salsa

- 1 cup cheddar cheese, shredded

Directions:

1. Add all ingredients to the slow cooker and stir well.

2. Cover slow cooker with lid and cook on low for 2 hours. Stir to mix.

3. Serve with fresh vegetables.

Nutrition:

- Calories 178 Fat 16.4 g Carbs 2.4 g Sugar 0.9 g Protein 6.1 g Cholesterol 46 mg

Easy Texas Dip

Preparation Time: 10 minutes

Cooking Time: 6 hours

Servings: 8

Ingredients:

- 1 ½ cups Velveeta cheese, cubed

- 2 cups fresh tomatoes, diced

- 4 oz. can green chilies, diced

- 1 large onion, chopped

Directions:

1. Add all ingredients into the slow cooker and stir well to combine.

2. Cover slow cooker with lid and cook on low for 6 hours.

3. Stir well and serve.

Nutrition:

- Calories 104 Fat 7.2 g Carbs 4.4 g Sugar 2.1 g Protein 6 g Cholesterol 22 mg

Cheese Chicken Dip

Preparation Time: 10 minutes

Cooking Time: 2 hours

Servings: 10

Ingredients:

- ½ cup bell peppers, chopped

- 1 cup chicken breast, cooked and shredded

- 12 oz. can tomato with green chilies

- ½ lb. cheese, cubed

Directions:

1. Add all ingredients into the slow cooker and stir well to combine.

2. Cover slow cooker with lid and cook on low for 2 hours.

3. Stir well and serve.

Nutrition:

- Calories 120 Fat 8 g Carbs 2 g Sugar 0.4 g Protein 10 g

Flavorful Mexican Cheese Dip

Preparation Time: 10 minutes

Cooking Time: 1 hour

Servings: 6

Ingredients:

- 1 tsp. taco seasoning

- ¾ cup tomatoes with green chilies

- 8 oz. Velveeta cheese, cut into cube

Directions:

1. Add cheese into the slow cooker. Cover and cook on low for 30 minutes. Stir occasionally.

2. Add taco seasoning and tomatoes with green chilies and stir well.

3. Cover again and cook on low for 30 minutes more.

4. Stir well and serve.

Nutrition:

- Calories 159 Fat 12.6 g Carbs 1.9 g Sugar 0.3 g Protein 9.6 g

Salsa Beef Dip

Preparation Time: 10 minutes

Cooking Time: 1 hour

Servings: 20

Ingredients:

- 32 Oz salsa

- 2 lbs. Velveeta cheese, cubed

- 2 lbs. ground beef

Directions:

1. Brown beef in a pan over medium heat. Drain well and transfer to the slow cooker.

2. Add cheese and salsa and stir well.

3. Cover slow cooker with lid and cook on high for 1 hour.

4. Stir well and serve.

Nutrition:

- Calories 279 Fat 17.9 g Carbs 3.4 g Sugar 1.6 g Protein 25.8 g Cholesterol 88 mg

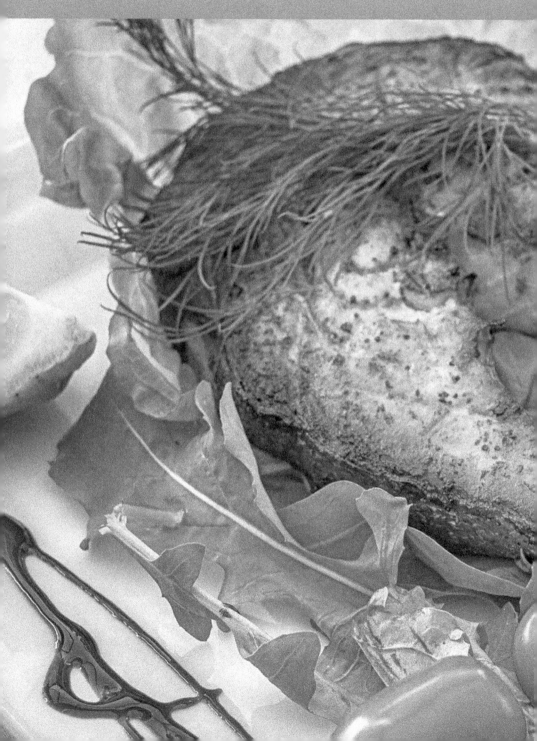

Fish & Seafood

Shrimp Scampi

Preparation Time: 5 minutes

Cooking Time: 2 hours and 30 minutes

Servings: 4

Ingredients:

- 1 pound wild-caught shrimps, peeled & deveined

- 1 tablespoon minced garlic

- 1 teaspoon salt

- ½ teaspoon ground black pepper

- 1/2 teaspoon red pepper flakes

- 2 tablespoons chopped parsley

- 2 tablespoons avocado oil

- 2 tablespoons unsalted butter

- 1/2 cup white wine

- 1 tablespoon lemon juice

- 1/4 cup chicken broth

- ½ cup grated parmesan cheese

Directions:

1. Place all the ingredients except for shrimps and cheese in a 6-quart slow cooker and whisk until combined.

2. Add shrimps and stir until evenly coated and shut with lid.

3. Plug in the slow cooker and cook for 1 hour and 30 minutes to 2 hours and 30 minutes at low heat setting or until cooked through.

4. Then top with parmesan cheese and serve.

Nutrition:

- Net Carbs 2 g Calories 234 Total Fat 14.7 g Saturated Fat 2 g Protein 23.3 g Carbs 2.1 g

  Fiber 0.1 g Sugar 2 g

Spicy Barbecue Shrimp

Preparation Time: 5 minutes

Cooking Time: 1 hour and 30 minutes

Servings: 6

Ingredients:

- 1 1/2 pounds large wild-caught shrimp, unpeeled
- 1 green onion, chopped
- 1 teaspoon minced garlic
- 1 ½ teaspoon salt
- ¾ teaspoon ground black pepper
- 1 teaspoon Cajun seasoning
- 1 tablespoon hot pepper sauce
- ¼ cup Worcestershire Sauce
- 1 lemon, juiced
- 2 tablespoons avocado oil
- 1/2 cup unsalted butter, chopped

Directions:

1. Place all the ingredients except for shrimps in a 6-quart slow cooker and whisk until mixed.

2. Plug in the slow cooker, then shut with lid and cook for 30 minutes at high heat setting.

3. Then take out ½ cup of this sauce and reserve.

4. Add shrimps to slow cooker.

Nutrition:

- Net Carbs 2.4 g Calories 321 Total Fat 21.4 g Saturated Fat 10.6 g Protein 27.3 g

  Carbs 4.8 g Fiber 2.4 g Sugar 1.2 g

Lemon Dill Halibut

Preparation Time: 5 minutes

Cooking Time: 2 hours

Servings: 2

Ingredients:

- 12-ounce wild-caught halibut fillet

- 1 teaspoon salt

- ½ teaspoon ground black pepper

- 1 1/2 teaspoon dried dill

- 1 tablespoon fresh lemon juice

- 3 tablespoons avocado oil

Directions:

1. Cut an 18-inch piece of aluminum foil, place halibut fillet in the middle and then season with salt and black pepper.

2. Whisk together remaining ingredients, drizzle this mixture over halibut, then crimp the edges of foil and place it into a 6-quart slow cooker.

3. Plug in the slow cooker, shut with lid and cook for 1 hour and 30 minutes or 2 hours at high heat setting or until cooked through.

4. When done, carefully open the crimped edges and check the fish, it should be tender and flaky.

5. Serve straightaway.

Nutrition:

- Net Carbs 0 g Calories 321.5 Total Fat 21.4 g Saturated Fat 7.2 g Protein 32.1 g Carbs 0 g

- Fiber 0 g Sugar 0.6 g

Coconut Cilantro Curry Shrimp

Preparation Time: 5 minutes

Cooking Time: 2 hours and 30 minutes

Servings: 4

Ingredients:

- 1 pound wild-caught shrimp, peeled and deveined

- 2 ½ teaspoon lemon garlic seasoning

- 2 tablespoons red curry paste

- 4 tablespoons chopped cilantro

- 30 ounces coconut milk, unsweetened

- 16 ounces water

Directions:

1. Whisk together all the ingredients except for shrimps and 2 tablespoons cilantro and add to a 4-quart slow cooker.

2. Plug in the slow cooker, shut with lid and cook for 2 hours at high heat setting or 4 hours at low heat setting.

3. Then add shrimps, toss until evenly coated and cook for 20 to 30 minutes at high heat settings or until shrimps are pink.

4. Garnish shrimps with remaining cilantro and serve.

Nutrition:

- Net Carbs 1.9 g Calories 160.7 Total Fat: 8.2 g Saturated Fat 8.1 g Protein 19.3 g

  Carbs 2.4 g Fiber 0.5 g Sugar 1.4 g

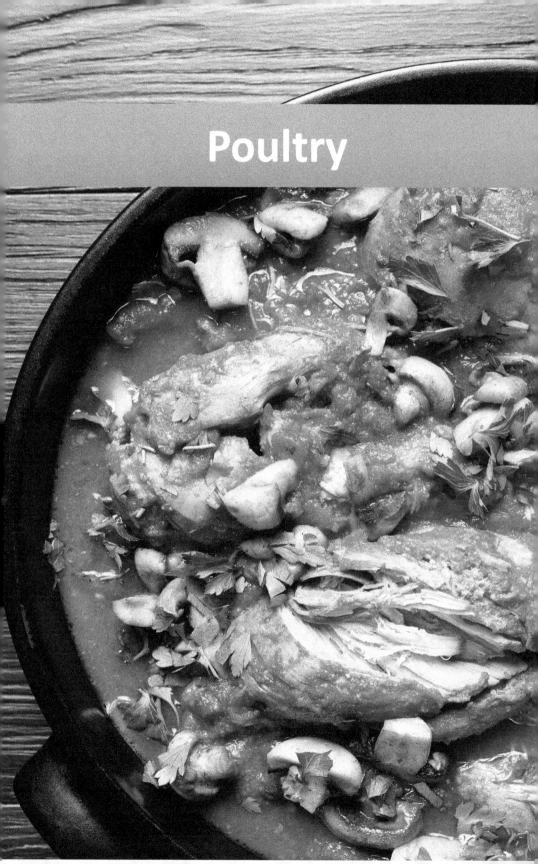

Poultry

Aromatic Jalapeno Wings

Preparation Time: 10 minutes

Cooking Time: 3 hours

Servings: 4

Ingredients:

- 1 jalapeño pepper, diced
- ½ cup of fresh cilantro, diced
- 3 tablespoon of coconut oil
- Juice from 1 lime
- 2 garlic cloves, peeled and minced
- Salt and black pepper ground, to taste
- 2 lbs. chicken wings
- Lime wedges, to serve
- Mayonnaise, to serve

Directions:

1. Start by throwing all the ingredients into the large bowl and mix well.
2. Cover the wings and marinate them in the refrigerator for 2 hours.
3. Now add the wings along with their marinade into the Crockpot.
4. Cover it and cook for 3 hours on Low Settings.
5. Garnish as desired.

6. Serve warm.

Nutrition:

- Calories 246 Total Fat 7.4 g Saturated Fat 4.6 g
  Cholesterol 105 mg Total Carbs 9.4 g

  Sugar 6.5 g Fiber 2.7 g Sodium 353 mg Potassium 529
  mg Protein 37.2 g

Turkey Meatballs

Preparation Time: 10 minutes

Cooking Time: 6 hours

Servings: 4

Ingredients:

- 1 lb. turkey meat, ground
- 1 yellow onion, minced
- 4 garlic cloves, minced
- ¼ cup of parsley, chopped
- salt, and black pepper to taste
- 1 teaspoon of oregano, dried
- 1 egg, whisked
- ¼ cup of almond milk
- 2 teaspoon of coconut aminos

- 12 mushrooms, diced
- 1 cup of chicken stock
- 2 tablespoon of olive oil
- 2 tablespoons of butter

Directions:

1. Thoroughly mix turkey meat with onion, garlic, parsley, pepper, salt, egg, aminos, and oregano in a bowl.
2. Make 1-inch small meatballs out of this mixture.
3. Add these meatballs along with other ingredients into the Crockpot.
4. Cover it and cook for 6 hours on Low Settings.
5. Garnish as desired.
6. Serve warm.

Nutrition:

- Calories 293 Total Fat 16 g Saturated Fat 2.3 g Cholesterol 75 mg Total Carbs 5.2 g

  Sugar 2.6 g Fiber 1.9 g Sodium 386 mg Potassium 907 mg Protein 34.2 g

Barbeque Chicken Wings

Preparation Time: 10 minutes

Cooking Time: 3 hours

Servings: 4

Ingredients:

- 2 lbs. chicken wings
- 1/2 cup of water
- 1/2 teaspoon of basil, dried
- 3/4 cup of BBQ sauce
- 1/2 cup of lime juice
- 1 teaspoon of red pepper, crushed
- 2 teaspoons of paprika
- 1/2 cup of swerve
- Salt and black pepper- to taste
- A pinch cayenne peppers

Directions:

1. Start by throwing all the ingredients into the Crockpot and mix them well.
2. Cover it and cook for 3 hours on Low Settings.
3. Garnish as desired.
4. Serve warm.

Nutrition:

- Calories 457 Total Fat 19.1 g Saturated Fat 11 g Cholesterol 262 mg Total Carbs 8.9 g

  Sugar 1.2 g Fiber 1.7 g Sodium 557 mg Potassium 748 mg Protein 32.5 g

Saucy Duck

Preparation Time: 10 minutes

Cooking Time: 6 hours

Servings: 4

Ingredients:

- 1 duck, cut into small chunks
- 4 garlic cloves, minced
- 4 tablespoons of swerves
- 2 green onions, roughly diced
- 4 tablespoon of soy sauce
- 4 tablespoon of sherry wine
- 1/4 cup of water
- 1-inch ginger root, sliced
- A pinch salt
- black pepper to taste

Directions:

1. Start by throwing all the ingredients into the Crockpot and mix them well.
2. Cover it and cook for 6 hours on Low Settings.
3. Garnish as desired.
4. Serve warm.

Nutrition:

*   Calories 338 Total Fat 3.8 g Saturated Fat 0.7 g Cholesterol 22 mg Total Carbs 8.3 g

    Fiber 2.4 g Sugar 1.2 g Sodium 620 mg Potassium 271 mg Protein 15.4 g

Chicken Roux Gumbo

Preparation Time: 10 minutes

Cooking Time: 6 hours

Servings: 24

Ingredients:

*   1 lb. chicken thighs, cut into halves
*   1 tablespoon of vegetable oil
*   1 lb. smoky sausage, sliced, crispy, and crumbled.
*   Salt and black pepper- to taste

Aromatics:

- 1 bell pepper, diced
- 2 quarts' chicken stock
- 15 oz. canned tomatoes, diced
- 1 celery stalk, diced
- salt to taste
- 4 garlic cloves, minced
- 1/2 lbs. okra, sliced
- 1 yellow onion, diced
- a dash tabasco sauce

For the roux:

- 1/2 cup of almond flour
- 1/4 cup of vegetable oil
- 1 teaspoon of Cajun spice

Directions:

1. Start by throwing all the ingredients except okra and roux ingredients into the Crockpot.
2. Cover it and cook for 5 hours on Low Settings.
3. Stir in okra and cook for another 1 hour on low heat.
4. Mix all the roux ingredients and add them to the Crockpot.
5. Stir cook on high heat until the sauce thickens.
6. Garnish as desired.
7. Serve warm.

Nutrition:

- Calories 604 Total Fat 30.6 g Saturated Fat 13.1 g Cholesterol 131 mg Total Carbs 1.4 g

  Fiber 0.2 g Sugar 20.3 g Sodium 834 mg Potassium 512 mg Protein 54.6 g

Cider-Braised Chicken

Preparation Time: 10 minutes

Cooking Time: 5 hours

Servings: 2

Ingredients:

- 4 chicken drumsticks

- 2 tablespoon of olive oil

- ½ cup of apple cider vinegar

- 1 tablespoon of balsamic vinegar

- 1 chili pepper, diced

- 1 yellow onion, minced

- Salt and black pepper- to taste

Directions:

1. Start by throwing all the ingredients into a bowl and mix them well.
2. Marinate this chicken for 2 hours in the refrigerator.
3. Spread the chicken along with its marinade in the Crockpot.
4. Cover it and cook for 5 hours on Low Settings.
5. Garnish as desired.
6. Serve warm.

Nutrition:

- Calories 311 Total Fat 25.5 g Saturated Fat 12.4 g Cholesterol 69 mg Total Carbs 1.4 g

  Fiber 0.7 g Sugar 0.3 g Sodium 58 mg Potassium 362 mg Protein 18.4 g

Chunky Chicken Salsa

Preparation Time: 10 minutes

Cooking Time: 6 hours

Servings: 2

Ingredients:

- 1 lb. chicken breast, skinless and boneless

- 1 cup of chunky salsa

- 3/4 teaspoon of cumin

- A pinch oregano

- Salt and black pepper- to taste

Directions:

1. Start by throwing all the ingredients into the Crockpot and mix them well.

2. Cover it and cook for 6 hours on Low Settings.

3. Garnish as desired.

4. Serve warm.

Nutrition:

- Calories 541 Total Fat 34 g Saturated Fat 8.5 g Cholesterol 69 mg Total Carbs 3.4 g

  Fiber 1.2 g Sugar 1 g Sodium 547 mg Potassium 467 mg Protein 20.3 g

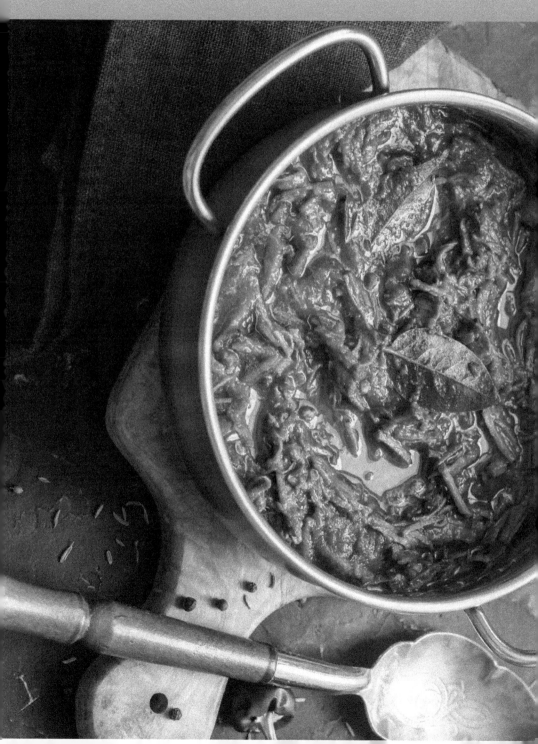

Lamb, Beef & Pork

Barbacoa Lamb

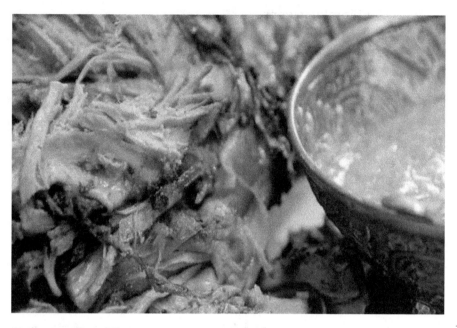

Preparation Time: 10 minutes

Cooking Time: Overnight (+) 6 hours – 25 minutes

Servings: 12

Ingredients:

- ¼ c. dried mustard

- 5 ½ lbs. leg of lamb - boneless

- 2 tbsp. of each:

- Smoked paprika

- Himalayan salt

- 1 tbsp. of each:

- Chipotle powder

- Dried oregano

- Ground cumin

- 1 c. water

Directions:

1. Combine the paprika, oregano, chipotle powder, cumin, and salt.

2. Cover the roast with the dried mustard, and sprinkle with the prepared spices. Arrange the lamb in the slow cooker, cover, and let it marinate in the refrigerator overnight.

3. In the morning, let the pot come to room temperature. Once you're ready to cook, just add the cup of water to the slow cooker on the high heat setting. Cook for six hours.

4. When done, remove all except for one cup of the cooking juices, and shred the lamb.

5. Using the rest of the cooking juices - adjust the seasoning as you desire, and serve

Nutrition:

- Calories 492 Net Carbs 1.2 g Fat 35.8 g Protein 37.5 g

Succulent Lamb

Preparation Time: 10 minutes

Cooking Time: 8 hours - 20 minutes

Servings: 6

Ingredients:

- ¼ c. olive oil
- 1 (2 lb.) leg of lamb
- 1 tbsp. maple syrup
- 2 tbsp. whole grain mustard
- 4 thyme sprigs
- 6-7 mint leaves
- ¾ t. of each:
- Dried rosemary
- Garlic
- Pepper & salt to taste

Directions:

1. Cut away the string/netting off the lamb. Slice three slits over the top.

2. Cover the meat with the oil and the rub (mustard, pepper, salt, and maple syrup). Push the rosemary and garlic into the slits.

3. Prepare on the low setting for seven hours. Garnish with the mint and thyme. Cook one more hour. Place on a platter and serve.

Nutrition:

- Calories 414 Net Carbs 0.3 g Fat 35.2 g Protein 26.7 g

BBQ Beef Burritos

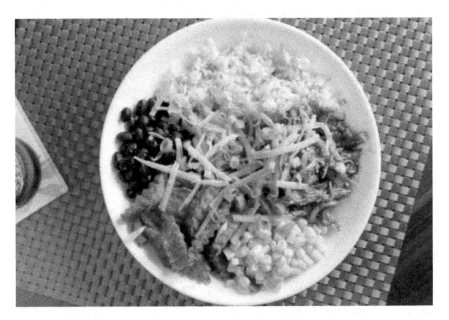

Preparation Time: 10 minutes

Cooking Time: 8 hours - 15 minutes

Servings: 4

Ingredients:

- 2 lb. top sirloin steak
- ½ t. black pepper
- 1 t. of each:
- Ground chipotle pepper – optional
- Cinnamon
- 2 t. of each:
- Sea salt
- Garlic powder
- 4 minced garlic cloves
- ½ white onion
- 2 bay leaves
- 1 c. of each:
- Chicken broth
- BBQ sauce – your favorite

Assembly Ingredients

- 1 ½ c. coleslaw mix
- 8 low-carb wraps
- ½ c. mayonnaise

Directions:

1. Pat the steak dry using some paper towels. Score with a sharp knife along the sides. Combine the seasonings and sprinkle on the meat.

2. Roughly chop the onion and mince the garlic and add to the crockpot. Pour in the broth. Add the steak and bay leaf. Secure the lid and cook eight hours on the low setting

3. When done, remove the steak and drain the juices. Arrange the beef, garlic, and onion back into the cooker and shred. Pour in the barbecue sauce and mix well.

4. Assemble the burritos using the beef fixings, a bit of slaw, and a dab of mayo.

Nutrition:

- Calories 750 Net Carbs 14 g Fat 48 g Protein 58 g

Cheeseburger & Bacon Pie

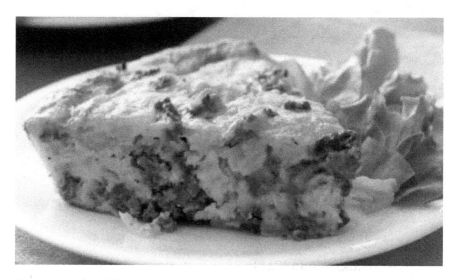

Preparation Time: 10 minutes

Cooking Time: 4 hours – 15 minutes

Servings: 8

Ingredients:

- 6 bacon slices – chopped
- 1 lb. ground beef
- 2 minced garlic cloves
- ¼ t. hot pepper flakes
- Pepper & Salt
- 6 large eggs
- 4 oz. softened cream cheese
- 1 ½ c. Mexican shredded cheese/shredded cheese

- Suggested to Use: 6-quart slow cooker

Directions:

1. Grease the cooker insert about 1/3 of the way up the sides.

2. Prepare the bacon until crispy in a skillet and drain on paper towels. Save the drippings and add the ground beef - cooking (med. heat) until browned.

3. Stir in the pepper flakes, garlic, pepper, and salt. Cook one minute and spread over the bottom of the cooker. Add ¾ of the bacon pieces and one cup of the cheese.

4. Whisk the eggs and cream cheese together until smooth. Scrape over the beef.

5. Prepare 3 ½ to 4 hours using the low-heat setting. The center should be just set.

6. Garnish with the rest of the cheese and secure the lid. Give it ten minutes to melt the cheese and sprinkle with the rest of the bacon. Serve and enjoy!

Nutrition:

- Calories 376 Fat 25.93 g Net Carbs 1.48 g Protein 28.21 g

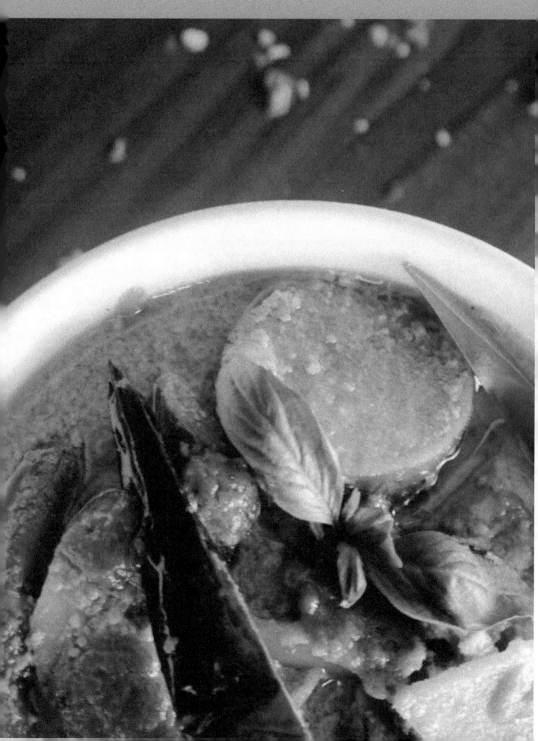

Lemon Asparagus

Preparation Time: 8 minutes

Cooking Time: 5 hours

Servings: 2

Ingredients:

- 8 oz. asparagus

- ½ cup butter

- juice of 1 lemon

- Zest of 1 lemon, grated

- ½ teaspoon turmeric

- 1 teaspoon rosemary, dried

Directions:

1. In your slow cooker, mix the asparagus with butter, lemon juice and the other ingredients and close the lid.
2. Cook the vegetables on Low for 5 hours. Divide between plates and serve.

Nutrition:

- calories 139 fat 4.6 g fiber 2.5 g carbs 3.3 g protein 3.5 g

Cheese Asparagus

Preparation Time: 10 minutes

Cooking Time: 3 hours

Servings: 4

Ingredients:

- 10 oz. asparagus, trimmed
- 4 oz. Cheddar cheese, sliced
- 1/3 cup butter, soft
- 1 teaspoon turmeric powder
- ½ teaspoon salt
- ¼ teaspoon white pepper

Directions:

1. In the slow cooker, mix the asparagus with butter and the other ingredients, put the lid on and cook for 3 hours on High.

Nutrition:

- calories 214 fat 6.2 g fiber 1.7 g carbs 3.6 g protein 4.2 g

Creamy Broccoli

Preparation Time: 15 minutes

Cooking Time: 1 hour

Servings: 4

Ingredients:

- ½ cup coconut cream
- 2 cups broccoli florets
- 1 teaspoon mint, dried
- 1 teaspoon garam masala

- 1 teaspoon salt

- 1 tablespoon almonds flakes

- ½ teaspoon turmeric

Directions:

1. In the slow cooker, mix the broccoli with the mint and the other ingredients.
2. Close the lid and cook vegetables for 1 hour on High.
3. Divide between plates and serve.

Nutrition:

- calories 102 fat 9 g fiber 1.9 g carbs 4.3 g protein 2.5 g

Curry Cauliflower

Preparation Time: 15 minutes

Cooking Time: 2.5 hours

Servings: 4

Ingredients:

- 1 ½ cup cauliflower, trimmed and florets separated

- 1 tablespoon curry paste

- ½ cup coconut cream

- 1 teaspoon butter

- ½ teaspoon garam masala

- ¾ cup chives, chopped

- 1 tablespoon rosemary, chopped

- 2 tablespoons Parmesan, grated

Directions:

1. In the slow cooker, mix the cauliflower with the curry paste and the other ingredients.
2. Cook the cauliflower for 2.5 hours on High.

Nutrition:

- Calories 146 Fat 4.3 g Fiber 1.9 g Carbs 5.7 g Protein 5.3 g

Garlic Eggplant

Preparation Time: 15 minutes

Cooking Time: 2 hours

Servings: 4

Ingredients:

- 1-pound eggplant, trimmed and roughly cubed

- 1 tablespoon balsamic vinegar

- 1 garlic clove, diced

- 1 teaspoon tarragon

- 1 teaspoon salt

- 1 tablespoon olive oil

- ½ teaspoon ground paprika

- ¼ cup of water

Directions:

1. In the slow cooker, mix the eggplant with the vinegar, garlic and the other ingredients, close the lid and cook on High for 2 hours.
2. Divide into bowls and serve.

Nutrition:

- Calories 132 Fat 2.8 g Fiber 4.7 g Carbs 8.5 g Protein 1.6 g

Coconut Brussels Sprouts

Preparation Time: 10 minutes

Cooking Time: 4 hours

Servings: 6

Ingredients:

- 2 cups Brussels sprouts, halved

- ½ cup of coconut milk

- 1 teaspoon garlic powder

- 1 teaspoon salt

- ½ teaspoon coriander, ground

- 1 teaspoon dried oregano

- 1 tablespoon balsamic vinegar

- 1 teaspoon butter

Directions:

1. Place Brussels sprouts in the slow cooker.

2. Add the rest of the ingredients, toss, close the lid and cook the Brussels sprouts for 4 hours on Low.
3. Divide between plates and serve.

Nutrition:
- Calories 128 Fat 5.6 g Fiber 1.7 g Carbs 4.4 g Protein 3.6 g

Cauliflower Pilaf with Hazelnuts

Preparation Time: 15 minutes

Cooking Time: 2 hours

Servings: 6

Ingredients:
- 3 cups cauliflower, chopped
- 1 cup chicken stock
- 1 teaspoon ground black pepper
- ½ teaspoon turmeric
- ½ teaspoon ground paprika
- 1 teaspoon salt
- 1 tablespoon dried dill
- 1 tablespoon butter
- 2 tablespoons hazelnuts, chopped

Directions:
1. Put cauliflower in the blender and blend until you get cauliflower rice.

2. Then transfer the cauliflower rice in the slow cooker.
3. Add ground black pepper, turmeric, ground paprika, salt, dried dill, and butter.
4. Mix up the cauliflower rice. Add chicken stock and close the lid.
5. Cook the pilaf for 2 hours on High.
6. Then add chopped hazelnuts and mix the pilaf well.

Nutrition:

- Calories 48 Fat 3.1 g Fiber 1.9 g Carbs 4.8 g Protein 1.6 g

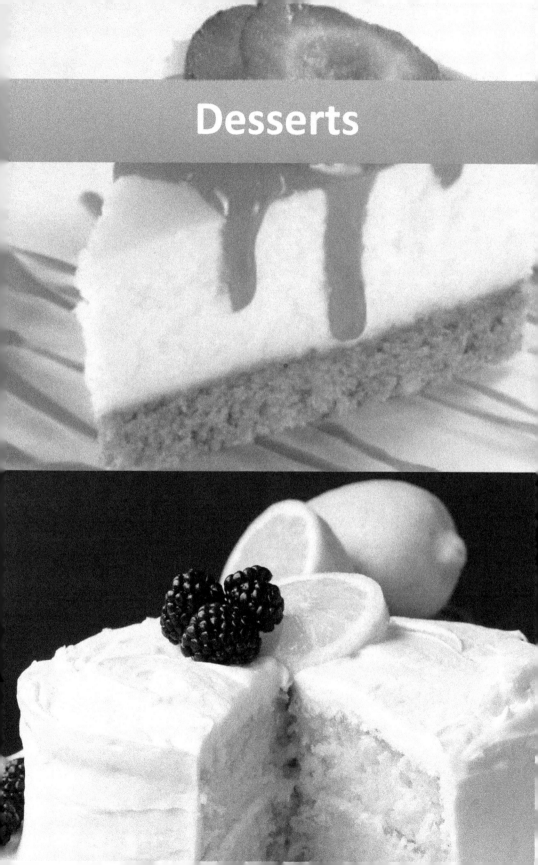

Desserts

Dark Chocolate Cake

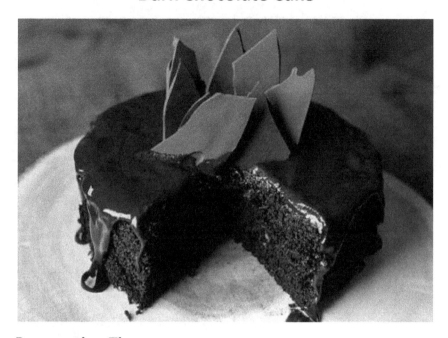

Preparation Time: 15 minutes

Cooking Time: 2 hours 30 minutes

Servings: 5

Ingredients:

- Almond flour – ½ cup plus 1 tbsp.

- Cocoa powder – ¼ cup

- Granular swerve – ¼ cup

- Baking powder – 1 tsp.

- Unflavored whey protein powder – 1 ½ tbsp.

- Salt – a pinch

- Melted butter – 3 tbsp.

- Vanilla extract – ½ tsp.

- Unsweetened almond milk – ¼ cup
- Chocolate chips – 2 tbsp., sugar-free
- Oil for the Crock-Pot

Directions:

1. Grease the Crock-Pot with oil.
2. Combine the protein powder, almond flour, sweetener, baking powder, salt, and cocoa powder.
3. Fold in the milk, butter, vanilla extract, and eggs until mixed. Mix in chips.
4. Add the batter into the Crock-Pot.
5. Cover and cook on high for 2 hours.
6. Turn off the heat and keep in the pot for 20 to 30 minutes more.
7. Slice and serve.

Nutrition:

- Calories 205 Fat 16.97 g Carbs 6.42 g Protein 7.37 g

Coconut Hot Chocolate

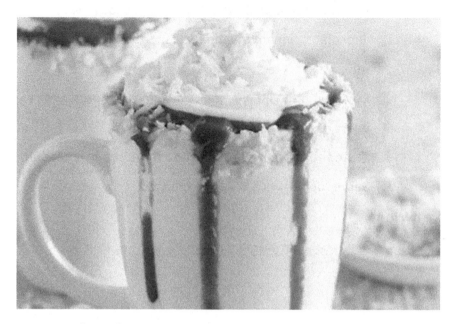

Preparation Time: 15 minutes

Cooking Time: 4 hours

Servings: 8

Ingredients:

- Full-fat coconut milk – 5 cups

- Heavy cream – 2 cups

- Vanilla extract – 1 tsp.

- Cocoa powder – 1/3 cup

- Dark chocolate – 3 ounces, no sugar added, chopped

- Cinnamon – ½ tsp.

- Stevia to taste

Directions:

1. Add the cream, milk, vanilla extract, cocoa powder, chocolate, cinnamon, and stevia to the Crock-Pot and mix.

2. Cover with the lid and cook on high for 4 hours. Whisk every 45 minutes.

3. Taste the hot chocolate and add more stevia if needed.

4. Serve topped with whipped cream.

Nutrition:

- Calories 339 Fat 30.3 g Carbs 7 g Protein 13.8 g

Lemon Cake

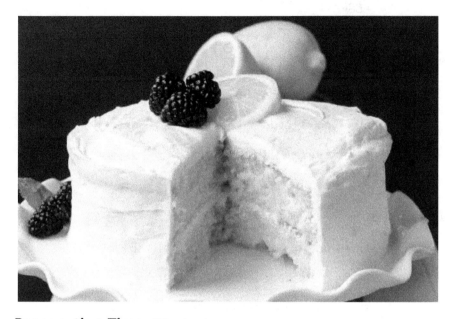

Preparation Time: 15 minutes

Cooking Time: 3 hours

Servings: 8

Ingredients:

- Coconut flour – ½ cup
- Almond flour – 1 ½ cups
- Baking powder – 2 tsp.
- Swerve – 6 tbsp.
- Xanthan gum – ½ tsp.
- Whipping cream – ½ cup
- Melted butter – ½ cup
- Zest of 2 lemons

- Juice of 2 lemons
- Eggs – 2

For the topping

- Boiling water – ½ cup
- Swerve – 3 tbsp.
- Lemon juice – 2 tbsp.
- Melted butter – 2 tbsp.

Directions:

1. Line the Crock-Pot with aluminum foil.
2. Make the cake: combine flours, baking powder, sweetener, and xanthan gum in a bowl. Whisk the butter and cream together, along with the zest, lemon juice, and egg in another bowl.
3. Combine all the ingredients and add to the cooker liner.
4. Make the topping: Mix all of the ingredients and pour over the cake in the pot. Cover and cook for 2 to 3 hours.
5. Serve warm.

Nutrition:

- Calories 350 Fat 32.6 g Carbs 5.2 g Protein 7.6 g

More Keto Recipes

Asparagus Bacon Bouquet

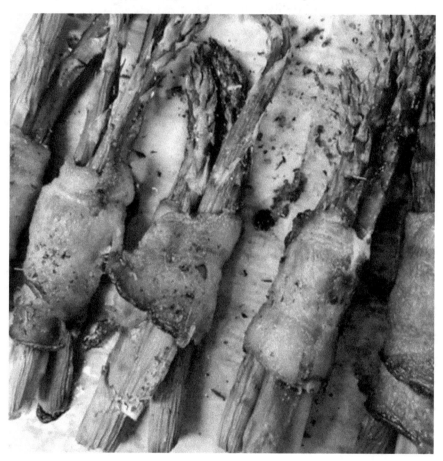

Preparation time: 15 minutes
Cooking time: 4 hours
Servings: 4

Ingredients:

- asparagus spears, trimmed

- slices bacon

- 1 tsp black pepper

- Extra virgin olive oil

Directions:

1   Coat slow cooker with extra virgin olive oil.
2   Slice spears in half, and sprinkle with black pepper
3   Wrap three spear halves with one slice bacon, and set inside the slow cooker.
4   Cook for 4 hours on medium.

Nutrition:

- Calories 345 Carbs 2 g Fat 27 g Protein 22 g Sodium 1311 mg Sugar 0 g

Madras Curry Chicken Bites

Preparation time: 15 minutes
Cooking time: 7 hours
Servings: 4
Ingredients:

- 1 lb. chicken breasts, skinless, boneless

- cloves garlic, grated

- 1 tsp ginger, grated

- 2 cups low-sodium chicken stock

- 2 lemons, juiced

- 1 tsp coriander, crushed

- 1 tsp cumin

- ½ tsp fenugreek

- 1 tbsp. curry powder

- ½ tsp cinnamon

- 1½ tsp salt

- 1 tsp black pepper

- Extra virgin olive oil

Directions:

1   Cube chicken breast into ½" pieces, and sprinkle with ½ tsp salt and ½ tsp black pepper.
2   Heat 3 tbsp. extra virgin olive oil in a skillet, add chicken breasts, and brown.
3   Place chicken breasts in a slow cooker.
4   Add chicken stock, garlic, lemon juice, spices, and salt.
5   Cook on low for 7 hours.

Nutrition:

- Calories 234 Carbs 3 g Fat 8 g Protein 38 g Sodium 782 mg Sugar 0 g

Spiced Jicama Wedges with Cilantro Chutney

Preparation time: 15 minutes
Cooking time: 4 hours
Servings: 8

Ingredients:

- 1 lb. jicama, peeled
- 1 tsp paprika
- ½ tsp dried parsley
- 2 tsp salt
- 2 tsp black pepper
- Extra virgin olive oil
- Cilantro Chutney
- 1 tsp dill chopped
- ¼ cup cilantro
- ½ tsp salt
- 1 tsp paprika
- 1tsp black pepper
- 2 lemons, juiced
- ¼ cup extra virgin olive oil

Directions:

1 Slice jicama into 1" wedges, and submerge in a bowl of cold water for 20 minutes.
2 Place the paprika, oregano, salt, black pepper in a bowl, and toss with jicama.
3 Add 5 tbsp. extra virgin olive oil into a bowl and coat well.
4 Place jicama in the slow cooker, and cook on high for 4 hours.

5   Combine Ingredients for chutney in blender, mix, and refrigerate until jicama wedges are ready to serve.

Nutrition:

- Calories 94 Carbs 5.2 g Fat 8 g Protein 1 g Sodium 879 mg Sugar 1 g

Teriyaki Chicken Wings

Preparation time: 15 minutes
Cooking time: 4 hours
Servings: 4
Ingredients:

- 2 lb. chicken wings

- 2 tsp ginger, grated

- cloves garlic, grated

- ¼ cup of soy sauce

- dates, pitted

- Extra virgin olive oil

Directions:

1   Processed the dates in a food processor along with 2 tbsp. soy sauce, and mix until pasty.
2   Combine ginger, garlic, soy sauce, and dates in a bowl, add chicken wings, coat, and refrigerate overnight.
3   Coat slow cooker with a little sesame oil, add chicken wings and cook on high for 4 hours.

Nutrition:

- Calories 354 Carbs 5.5 g Fat 16 g Protein 45 g Sodium 730 mg Sugar 0 g

Portabella Pizza Bites

Preparation time: 15 minutes
Cooking time: 5 hours
Servings: 8
Ingredients:

- Portabella Mushrooms

- ½ lb. ground pork

- 1 medium onion, diced

- cloves garlic, grated

- 2 cups crushed tomato

- ½ cup Mozzarella, shredded

- ¼ cup Parmesan

- ½ tsp oregano

- 1 tsp salt

- 1 tsp black pepper

- Garnish

- ½ cup parsley, chopped

Directions:

1   Coat 6 qt. slow cooker with extra virgin olive oil

2   Heat 3 tbsp. extra virgin olive oil in a skillet, add pork, brown.

3   Mix crushed tomato with salt, black pepper, oregano, parmesan, and garlic.

4   Spoon a little tomato-parmesan mixture into each mushroom, add a little ground pork, and sprinkle with Mozzarella.

5   Place each mushroom in a slow cooker. Cook pizza bites on medium for 5 hours.

6   Sprinkle a little parsley on top before serving.

Nutrition:

Calories 106 Carbs 5.6 g Fat 3 g Protein 13 g Sodium 421 mg Sugar 2 g

Candied Walnuts

Preparation time: 15 minutes
Cooking time: 2 hours & 30 minutes
Servings: 16
Ingredients:

- ½ cup unsalted butter

- 1-pound walnuts

- ½ cup Splenda, granular

- 1½ teaspoons ground cinnamon

- ¼ teaspoon ground allspice

- ¼ teaspoon ground ginger

- 1/8 teaspoon ground cloves

Directions:

1. Set a slow cooker on high and preheat for about 15 minutes. Add butter and walnuts and stir to combine.
2. Add the Splenda and stir to combine well. Cook, covered, for about 15 minutes.
3. Uncover the slow cooker and stir the mixture. Set to cook on low, uncovered, within 2 hours, stirring occasionally.
4. Transfer the walnuts to a bowl. In another small bowl, mix spices.
5. Sift spice mixture over walnuts and toss to coat evenly. Set aside to cool before serving.

Nutrition:

- Calories 227 Carbohydrates 10.5g Protein 6.9g Fat 22.5g Sugar 7g Sodium 42mg Fiber 2.1g

Conclusion

Now you can cook healthier meals for yourself, your family, and your friends that will get your metabolism running at the peak of perfection and will help you feel healthy, lose weight, and maintain a healthy balanced diet. A new diet isn't so bad when you have so many options from which to choose. You may miss your carbs, but with all these tasty recipes at your fingertips, you'll find them easily replaced with new favorites.

You will marvel at how much energy you have after sweating though the first week or so of almost no carbs. It can be a challenge, but you can do it! Pretty soon you won't miss those things that bogged down your metabolism as well as your thinking and made you tired and cranky. You will feel like you can rule the world and do anything, once your body is purged of heavy carbs and you start eating things that rejuvenate your body. It is worth the few detox symptoms when you actually start enjoying the food you are eating.

A Keto diet isn't one that you can keep going on and off. It will take your body some time to get adjusted and for ketosis to set in. This process could take anywhere between two to seven days. It depends on the level of activity, your body type and the food that you are eating.

There are various mobile applications that you can make use of to track your carbohydrate intake. There are paid and free applications as well. These apps will help you in keeping a track of your total carbohydrate and fiber intake. However, you won't be able to track your net carb intake. MyFitnessPal is one of the popular apps. You just need to open the app store on your smartphone, and you can select an app from the various apps that are available.

The amount of weight that you will lose will depend on you. If you add exercise to your daily routine, then the weight loss will be greater. If you cut down on foods that stall weight loss, then this will speed up the process. For instance, completely cutting out things like artificial sweeteners, dairy and wheat products and other related products will definitely help in speeding up your weight loss. During the first two weeks of the Keto diet, you will end up losing all the excess water weight. Ketosis has a diuretic effect on the body, and you might end up losing a couple of pounds within the first few days of this diet. After this, your body will adapt itself to burn fats to generate energy, instead of carbs.

Now you have everything you need to break free from a dependence on highly processed foods, with all their dangerous additives that your body interprets as toxins. Today, when you want a sandwich for lunch, you'll roll the meat in Swiss cheese or a lettuce leaf and won't miss the bread at all, unless that is, you've made up the Keto bread recipe you discovered in this book! You can still enjoy your favorite pasta dishes, even taco salad, but without the grogginess in the afternoon that comes with all those unnecessary carbs.

So, energize your life and sustain a healthy body by applying what you've discovered. You don't have to change everything at once. Just start by adopting a new recipe each week that sounds interesting to you. Gradually, swap out less-than-healthy options for ingredients and recipes from this book that will promote your well-being.

Each time you make a healthy substitution or try a new ketogenic recipe, you can feel proud of yourself; you are actually taking good care of your mind and body. Even before you start to experience the benefits of a ketogenic lifestyle, you can feel good because you are choosing the best course for your life.

Thanks for reading.

Conversion Tables

Volume Equivalents (Liquid)

US STANDARD	US STANDARD (OUNCES)	METRIC (APPROXIMATE)
2 tablespoons	1 fl. oz.	30 mL
¼ cup	2 fl. oz.	60 mL
½ cup	4 fl. oz.	120 mL
1 cup	8 fl. oz.	240 mL
1½ cups	12 fl. oz.	355 mL
2 cups or 1 pint	16 fl. oz.	475 mL
4 cups or 1 quart	32 fl. oz.	1 L
1 gallon	128 fl. oz.	4 L

Volume Equivalents (Dry)

US STANDARD	METRIC (APPROXIMATE)
¼ teaspoon	1 mL
½ teaspoon	2 mL
1 teaspoon	5 mL
1 tablespoon	15 mL
¼ cup	59 mL
cup	79 mL
½ cup	118 mL
1 cup	177 mL

Oven Temperatures

FAHRENHEIT (F)	CELSIUS (C) (APPROXIMATE)
250°F	120 °C
300°F	150°C
325°F	165°C
350°F	180°C
375°F	190°C
400°F	200°C
425°F	220°C
450°F	230°C

Weight Equivalents

US STANDARD	METRIC (APPROXIMATE)
½ ounce	15 g
1 ounce	30 g
2 ounces	60 g
4 ounces	115 g
8 ounces	225 g
12 ounces	340 g
16 ounces or 1 pound	455 g

CPSIA information can be obtained
at www.ICGtesting.com
Printed in the USA
BVHW081554260521
608179BV00004B/879